Type Two Diabetes

Vanessa B. Jackson

West Chester University – Graduate School

Illustrator: Cover Image 2021

Tom Centola

TomCentola-illustrations.com

ABSTRACT

The book investigates Type 2 Diabetes Mellitus (T2DM), how it develops, and the effect of Diabetes within the body. The bulk of the research has been retrieved from EBSCO and Credo, the leading provider of research databases, e-journals, magazines, etc. In addition, I conducted an exclusive interview with someone who was recently diagnosed with Type 2 diabetes; his real-time testimony will convey 5% of this research. The study will reveal the differences between Type 1 diabetes—which is often genetic, and Type 2—which is often a result of obesity, an unhealthy, unbalanced diet—and an inactive lifestyle. Together we will discover why some people do not understand the differences between the two disorders—and why heaps of people find it difficult to change their diet and/or lifestyle to help alleviate maladies. The end of the book offers cognitive therapy exercises for your spiritual growth and development.

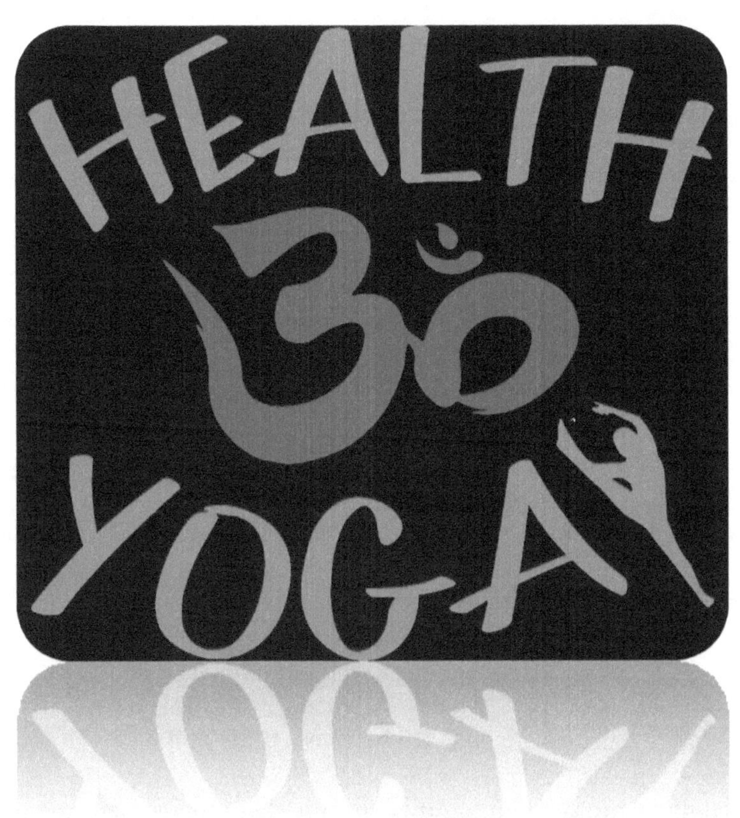

HEALTH
ॐ
YOGA

Type Two Diabetes

There are heaps of people in our society who cannot grasp the importance of a healthy diet and active lifestyle. In today's world, people want to eat-eat-eat, not realizing or understanding the effect of an unhealthy and unbalanced diet. Many people eat when they are bored, depressed, stressed, happy, or just because they can—and this is where health-related problems are created. Food is delicious, and food is an essential product needed to survive, but too much of anything isn't good for you! When people overconsume food for an extended amount of time and lack an active lifestyle, Type 2 Diabetes is often the adverse effect of that action. Note, it usually takes years of eating poorly before a person's health is affected.

Today we will discuss Type 2 Diabetes Mellitus and how the foods we eat have a significant role in developing this chronic disorder. Statistics have proven that Diabetes is on the rise in the United States. "Nearly 1.6 million Americans are diagnosed with Diabetes every year" (American Diabetes Association, para. 1). The question is, is there something society can do about this soaring predicament? According to the American Diabetes Association, people can prevent and/or delay Type Two Diabetes Mellitus (T2DM). "That's right, making changes to the way you eat, increasing physical activity levels and getting early treatment could return blood sugar levels to a normal range" (American Diabetes Association, 2001, para. 1-2). If this is the case, why are so many people refusing to find integrative ways to control health conditions? When doctors and patients choose integrative techniques, they consider the lifestyle and activities of the person. They work on treating the whole person; it's a mind, body, and soul experience. Altering unhealthy habits could potentially change your life!

Diabetes is a chronic disease, meaning ongoing; it doesn't cause immediate death, and disorders can last throughout a lifetime. "Chronic diseases are medical conditions that last one year or more and require continuing medical attention" (CDC & Prevention, 2021, para 1). It is believed that it's easier to take prescription drugs than to change one's diet and lifestyle; after all, change is hard and can be impossible for some. However, many people will get fed up with prescribed medications and eventually seek holistic approaches to decrease illnesses. Some people need time to build mental strength to make appropriate and essential lifestyle changes. According to Yi-Jen et al., "The global prevalence of age-standardized type 2 diabetes mellitus (T2DM) was predicted to be 9.3% (463 million people) in 2019, and it is projected to rise to 10.2% (578 million) and 10.9% (700 million) by 2030 and 2045, respectively. Diabetes can lead to several complications, including damage to the eyes, heart, kidneys, nerves, and blood vessels, and approximately 50% of DM patients die of cardiovascular disease. The World Health Organization (WHO) warns that DM will be the seventh leading cause of death in 2030. The risk factors associated with T2DM are multiplex but largely comprise rapid increases in overweight, high body mass index, less physical activity, inactive lifestyles, and high frequencies of high fat intake." (Yi-Jen et al., 2021, p.1 para 1).

With statistical analysis such as this, you may wonder why people have to experience the worst before making lifestyle changes? The answer is simple, eating healthy and being active takes discipline, hard work, and dedication. This type of self-care often takes time to develop. The brain must be rewired; patterns and habits create Neuroplasticity, which is the brain's ability to rewire itself, literally changing how we view the world around us and the activities we do throughout our daily lives. The power to create change comes from within, and it starts with a strong desire to want more out of life.

According to Ratnesh et al., "Living successfully with T2DM requires lifelong discipline and commitment, which could be very demanding, stressful, and depressing. Diabetes Distress (DD) refers to psychological distress specific to people living with Diabetes. It can encompass a wide range of emotions, such as feeling overwhelmed by the demands of self-management required through adherence to diet, exercise, and medications. They may worry about existing or future complications, be fearful of Hypoglycemia, and harbor feelings of guilt or shame, notably in relation to obesity or lifestyle. Diabetes distress lowers the motivation for self-care, often leading to decreased physical and emotional wellbeing" (Ratnesh et al., 2020, para. 2-4). Fear is a lier—it's fear that often stops people from advancing in life. Here is where emotional support from family and friends and guidance from qualified doctors and practitioners comes into play. People often need motivation and inspiration; thus, our influences and environments could determine our overall outcome in life. Indeed, we are the company we keep, and many people throughout the world realize this essential fact—and they are choosing their company wisely.

According to Afaya et al., "Diabetes mellitus is a complex disease that affects many organ systems, leading to concerns about deteriorating population health status and ever-increasing healthcare expenditure. Many people with diabetes do not achieve optimal glycaemic control and other metabolic indices, leading to a heightened risk of developing complications. Adequate knowledge of diabetes complications is a prerequisite for risk-factor reduction and prevention of the consequences of the disease" (Afaya et al., 2020 p. 1, para. 1). Knowledge and health literacy are crucial components to controlling maladies. Regrettably, many old-school doctors and some new school physicians do not take the time to ensure their patients fully understand their diagnoses. Thus, patients may not be aware of how to restore their health and wellbeing.

Moreover, when I was talking with my neighbor, he informed me that he has Diabetes, and my first response was, are you type one or type two? And to my surprise, he wasn't sure which type he had. Thus, out of curiosity, I asked (I'll call

my neighbor Mike) if he always had diabetes and when he was diagnosed. Mike

informed me that the diagnosis was given as he aged; this information told me that

he had Type 2 diabetes; it wasn't genetic but created by lifestyle and diet. I asked

him about his diet and how often he exercised, and the conversation blossomed

from there. We will hear Mike's testimony later in this paper.

Unlike Type 2 Diabetes Mellitus—Type 1 diabetes isn't created by obesity

and lifestyle but is a result of a pancreas malfunction; this is often genetic, meaning

the person was born with the disorder—or a serious accident could have

ruined/damages the pancreas. When the pancreas isn't functioning properly, it

produces little to no insulin, which causes Type 1 Diabetes. According to Khan,

"Type 1 diabetes is common in children and young adults. The body is unable to

produce insulin, so insulin is injected daily. This condition is caused by

autoimmune destruction of the pancreatic islets beta cells. Several factors can play

a role in type 1 diabetes, such as environment, inheritance, genetic susceptibility,

viral infections, and autoimmune factors" (Khan, 2008). Insulin is an essential

hormone that regulates and controls blood sugar levels. Without this regulation, the

body will go into hyperglycemic shock, which is dangerously high blood sugar

levels, which could lead to a coma. So, as you can see, there is a vast difference

between Type 1 and Type 2 diabetes. Type 2 *can* be reversed with proper diet and exercise; however, Type 1 has no cure, a damaged pancreas will always be damaged. Type 1 diabetes is insulin-dependent. Type 2 uses drug therapy to rid the body of excessive sugar in the blood; it's insulin-resistant.

Why is it that Mike and so many other people like him are benighted to their diagnosis? Could it be that many physicians spend very little time discussing diagnoses with their patients? Though the doctor or nurse will give their patients an informational brochure to read, maybe this isn't enough. Most patients need a thorough conversation about their diagnosis, and without this detailed talk, some patients become uninformed of their malady. A study conducted by Afaya et al., aimed to evaluate the knowledge of chronic complications of diabetes among persons living with Type 2 Diabetes Mellitus. The majority of participants (54.1%) had inadequate knowledge, and 45.9% had adequate knowledge of diabetes complications (Afaya, para. 1 & 3). This article supports the notion that over 50% of people diagnosed with Type 2 diabetes do not have adequate knowledge and/or understanding of their malady. And when people lack understanding of their illnesses, they often do not know efficient ways to keep their disease under control.

However, when the person becomes aware and starts to understand how their disease works, they can develop skills and healthy habits to decrease symptoms. Indeed, medication combined with a healthy and active lifestyle has been proven to reduce diabetic symptoms significantly—and for some people, they were able to reduce their A1C levels. Here's an urgent notice, exercise prompts muscles to absorb sugar from the bloodstream; hence, blood sugar levels drop more rapidly with physical activity. Many people with diabetes have been informed that physical activity is an essential part of their care plan; however, the explanation of what is happening within the body is often omitted; this is pertinent information and should be conveyed to patients. Adequate information could allow someone who is struggling with their diagnosis to see things more clearly.

You may be wondering what does A1C detect? According to the Center for Disease Control (CDC), "When sugar enters your bloodstream, it attaches to hemoglobin, a protein in your red blood cells. Everybody has some sugar attached to their hemoglobin, but people with higher blood sugar levels have more. The A1C test measures the percentage of your red blood cells that have sugar-coated hemoglobin" (CDC, 2018, para. 3). People who see their primary care physician (PCP) annually often receive a warning from their doctors about their A1C levels. A simple blood test (finger prick) can deliver these results. Early detection and preventative care are essential for a healthy body. According to the CDC, "The normal range for A1C is below 5.7% — and 5.7% - 6.4% is considered prediabetes. To be diagnosed with Type 2 Diabetes, the A1C level must be 6.5% or above (CDC, para. 7). If you haven't already done so, maybe you can schedule a yearly appointment with a physician. Early detection for *any* illness has the power to save lives. According to the CDC, "people should consider getting a baseline A1C test done if they are over the age of 45—or overweight" (CDC, para. 4).

When we see our PCP regularly, they may run standard tests to ensure we are in optimum health; and once we reach a specific age, doctors search for aged-acquired illness. Early detection is essential in saving lives. Furthermore, preventative care could delay or stop certain maladies. Preventative care is measures taken to prevent and or reduce illnesses. Preventive care includes vaccines and routine testing. In addition, preventative care starts from within. I'm talking about the foods we put into our bodies, activity levels, environmental factors, stressors, smoking, alcohol, etc.

Our diet and Activities of Daily Living (ADL) decide how our cells and molecules react. When our bodies have too much oxidation, the cells within our bodies overreact, creating disease and/or inflammation. Let's take, for example, antioxidants—like Diabetes; many people do not know precisely what antioxidants are. Yes, the name is familiar, but how many people are knowledgeable about what it means and the effect antioxidants have on the body?

According to Medical News Today (MNT), "Antioxidants are substances that can prevent or slow damage to cells caused by free radicals—which are unstable molecules that the body produces as a reaction to environmental factors and the foods we eat, including alcohol and cigarettes. The sources of antioxidants can be natural or artificial. Certain fruits and vegetables are thought to be rich in antioxidants. The body also produces some antioxidants, known as endogenous antioxidants. Antioxidants that come from outside the body are called exogenous" Medical News Today, 2021. para. 1-3). In a nutshell, antioxidants fight to prevent or slow down the production of damaged cells; hence, diseases are reduced. Antioxidants are lean, mean, free-radical fighting machines.

Free radicals damage our bodies, and antioxidants work to protect us from them. According to MNT, "Free radicals are waste substances produced by cells as the body processes food and reacts to our environment. If the body cannot process and remove free radicals efficiently, **oxidative stress** can result; this can harm cells and body function" (MNT, para. 4). Oxidative stress is a by-product of free radicals, and Anti**oxidants** are an essential element needed to stop/slow **oxidation/free-radicals** in its tract. This is the first line of defense of preventative care; it comes from within. If we increase the number of fruits and vegetables we put into our bodies, we can slow down and/or reduce illnesses. And if we add a clean environment, reduce the amount of stress we endure, and work out daily, our bodies become barriers against disease and infections. Please note that unhealth, processed, high-calorie foods, alcohol, and tobacco increase free radicals; these items must be consumed moderately.

Now when we go to the market to purchase groceries, we will be aware of the word antioxidant, and we will know the meaning of the word and its effect on our bodies. Here's another excerpt regarding antioxidants and free radicals; according to The Gale Encyclopedia of Diets, "The role of antioxidants in the body is complex and not completely understood. Antioxidants combine with free radicals so that the free radicals cannot react with, or oxidize, other molecules. In this way, antioxidants help slow or prevent damage to cells. Antioxidant enzymes present in the body also work to prevent oxidation. Damage caused by free radicals is thought to cause or contribute to cardiovascular disease, cancer, Alzheimer's disease, age-related changes in vision, and other signs of aging" (The Gale Encyclopedia of Diets, para. 2). Hence, antioxidants to the rescue. What a joy to know that we can reduce free radicals and oxidation by simply eating healthy foods. Once we know better, we can do better.

Let's discuss my neighbor Mike. Mike is in his mid-50's, and he has a semi-active career; every so often, he will go to the gym or play basketball. He also runs errands and helps the elderly on his days off, so he's a pretty active person. Mike's issue isn't laziness but the food he eats. He's from the south and loves a hearty meal, though he will try to eat healthy now and then. Mike only cooks with olive oil, which we know is a heart-healthy oil, but Mike uses a lot of it when he cooks. And let's remember, too much of anything isn't a good thing. He also loves carbs/starches and enjoys fried-battered foods. He sometimes drinks zero-calorie beverages, which use artificial sweeteners to give the product its sweet taste. Mike enjoys fruity cocktails; thus, he limits his alcohol intake. In addition, Mike loves water and will eat fruits and vegetables from time to time. This information tells me that Mike is trying to live a healthy lifestyle—and has made some adjustments to his diet. Withal, Mike's A1C levels are above 6.5%, but the number is decreasing—he's on the road to recovery, and I am very proud of him.

Today, Mike better understands his disorder, and he is aware of what is needed to bring his A1C levels down. He makes a habit of checking his glucose levels before and after meals, and he's working on losing a few extra pounds, mainly around the abdominal area. Mike understands that if his sugar levels are high after a meal, a simple walk and a few strength-building exercises will rapidly reduce his blood sugar levels. Mike's a trooper; he's adamant about controlling his disease! I will continue to work with Mike and keep track of his astounding progress.

As we know, healing takes time, we cannot reverse health conditions overnight, but we can decide to change our diet and lifestyle overnight—it starts with a desire to change one's current situation. Remember, "the day you plant the seed—isn't the day you eat the fruit—be patient and trust the process" (Fabienne Fredrickson). Once we make a sincere decision to create a new life, nothing or no one can stop us! Willpower and perseverance often take us to new and exciting places.

In today's world, willpower is considered a superpower. There are so many unhealthy fast-food options available to use—and as a result, diabetes prevalence is increasing. Regrettably, Type 2 Diabetes isn't only affecting middle-aged women and men; it's also affecting children and adolescence; this is because childhood obesity is on the rise. Americans live in a society where almost all fast-food choices can be supersized, and many kids and adults are taking the supersized options. Of course, discipline is the key, but responsible parenting and providing balance in your child's diet are also essential. The child often doesn't know better; however, the parents do. Thankfully many elementary schools and high schools are implementing health and wellness in the classrooms. According to Castorani et al., "Type 2 diabetes (T2D) is an emerging health risk in obese children and adolescents. Environmental factors, including lack of physical activity, inadequate nutritional intake, inactive lifestyle, and genetic factors, contribute to this global epidemic" (Castorani, Polidori, Giannini, Blasetti, & Chiarelli, 2020, p. 1, para. 1).

Genetic factors regarding Type 2 diabetes includes learned eating patterns and the way families prepare meals. Suppose a child's immediate family eats unhealthy foods and cook meals high in calories, fats and sugars—with little to no fruits and vegetables—the child will likely adopt the same eating and cooking patterns. Nonetheless, education and a clear understanding of free radicals and antioxidants can break learned genetic habits. And when people understand the effect food has on the body, they often think twice before they supersize that value meal.

Have you noticed that a garden salad cost more than a burger, fries, and a sugary soft drink? This is a major concern for many Americans and a fundamental reason why obesity and health conditions are growing in the United States. As we all know, fruits and veggies are grown naturally *and* can be grown in abundance, so why do they cost more? Why do a burger, French fries, and a sugary soft drink—that doesn't grow in abundance and need to be processed, meaning artificial products cost less? These are the things that make me go, umm! It literally puzzles me. Having a burger and fries occasionally is a spectacular treat, but for a healthy body, these types of foods must be limited but often aren't because they are easy to come by, taste delicious, and cost less. These types of unhealthy eating choices aid in the growing number of Type 2 diabetes in children.

According to Berstein H & Berstein L, "The number of children, and adults with Type 2 Diabetes Mellitus has been growing considerably in recent years. This condition used to be known as "adult-onset diabetes" because it was so uncommon among children and adolescents. Since the 1990s, however, more cases of type 2 diabetes mellitus are being diagnosed in children than ever before" (Berstein H &

Berstein L, 2019, para. 1). Why is it that so many children are developing type two diabetes? There are many factors involved with this situation, but I'm sure key factors include poor diet and reduced physical activity.

Berstein & Berstein goes on to say, "Type 2 diabetes is the most common form of Diabetes mellitus in the United States, affecting more than 25 million people. Both type 1 and type 2 diabetes cause high amounts of sugar (glucose) to circulate in the blood. Insulin produced by the pancreas is required to move sugar from the blood into the body's cells, where the sugar is used to create energy. People with type 1 diabetes do not make enough or any insulin. People with type 2 diabetes initially make plenty of insulin, but their cells are resistant to the action of insulin (insulin resistance). The cells do not respond properly, and high levels of sugar build up in their blood. Persistently high blood sugars make it hard for the body to fight infections and, over time, damage nerves and blood vessels, causing problems with the heart, brain, eyes, kidneys, feet, as well as other parts of the body" (Bernstein H, & Berstein L, 2019, para. 2-4). As we can see, Diabetes Mellitus is a serious disorder and can lead to other health conditions; thus, it should be taken seriously.

Bernstein's article backs up my statement regarding lack of activity by saying, "Some people believe Type 2 Diabetes in kids may be related to changes in children's diets, activity levels, and weights. Children, like adults, are eating more calories than ever before. At the same time, children are getting less exercise, both in school and at home. Higher calorie diets and less exercise together mean more children are overweight. It is now estimated that one child out of every three in the United States is at least somewhat overweight" (Bernstein, para. 5). Maybe society will get creative and find ways to get children outdoors. A walk is nice, but a run, bike ride, skating, hiking, etc., is better. Maybe we can start out walking and advance to more intense forms of physical activities; here is where the heart and lungs advance. Of course, the person must be healthy enough to do physical activities, so please speak with your PCP before starting any exercise regimen.

Many people do not develop health-related symptoms right away; Diabetes can go undetected for years; however, a simple blood test can keep people up to date with their A1C levels. According to Bernstein, "Most people with type 2 diabetes have no signs or symptoms, or their symptoms are so mild that they are not even noticed. Some people do have symptoms, which may include increased thirst, increased hunger, increased urination, extreme fatigue, blurred vision, or cuts and sores that do not heal well. Some adolescents with type 2 diabetes, particularly those who are overweight, have areas of dark, thickened, velvety skin in the folds of the neck or abdomen, under the arms, inside the elbow, or on the inner thighs. This condition, called acanthosis nigricans, is associated with persistently high insulin levels in the blood and marked insulin resistance. High blood pressure, abnormal cholesterol and triglyceride blood levels, and irregular menstrual periods may be signs of type 2 diabetes" (Bernstein 2020, para. 7-9). Heaps of people experience signs of physical distress, but we often dismiss the symptoms—oblivious to what our bodies are trying to communicate to us. We sometimes feel sluggish or sick after eating a particular meal or drinking specific drinks; this too is a signal from our body. Maybe we can raise our awareness and pay more attention to what is going on within.

You may be wondering what foods are safe and effective for diabetics? Well, there are plenty of foods you can eat, and some unhealthy ones too. However, unhealthy foods must be eaten in moderation. According to Healthy Eating for T2D, "Eat a well-balanced diet that emphasizes fruit, vegetables, whole grains, and lean protein, while watching total calories and getting regular exercise. What you choose to eat daily is up to you, but the overall goal is to maintain a healthy weight and exercise regularly. You should also focus on keeping your blood sugar levels close to normal to prevent long-term complications of Diabetes and avoid the short-term consequences of low blood sugar" (Healthy Eating for T2D, 2019, para. 1-2). When monitoring our glucose levels daily, we are staying proactive in the fight against diabetes.

According to the CDC, "Normal blood glucose ranges between 70-140 milligrams per deciliter (mg/dL) (Health line, 2021). When Mike and I first started discussing diabetes, he wasn't sure what the standard levels were. He recently had a reading of 130 mg/dL after a meal and thought the results were high; however, those numbers were ideal after eating. I politely reviewed the normal blood glucose range with Mike—and he realized he's right on track. Sometimes people just need a little reinforcement or someone to boost their memory about their malady. Many doctors and practitioners recommend diabetes support groups because peer counseling has a way of keeping people on track and up to date!

Keeping track of glucose levels can save people from unnecessary complications. For example, when a person has low blood sugar, which is called **Hypoglycemia,** they may experience weakness, dizziness, anxieties, headaches, paleness of skin, and even loss of consciousness. Remember, sugar/carbohydrates are the body's primary energy source; without them, the body doesn't operate as it should. A Diabetic must check their sugar levels daily to ensure their levels aren't too low or too high. High blood sugar is known as **Hyperglycemia**. Hyperglycemia may cause dry mouth, fatigue, blurred vision, seizures, and could even lead to a diabetic coma. So, you see, staying on top of Diabetes and checking sugar levels is imperative.

According to Hypoglycemia, "When blood sugar levels are low, the body tries to normalize levels by releasing epinephrine, a hormone that not only increases the heart rate and blood pressure but also speeds up metabolism so that more glucose is released. High epinephrine levels can result in sudden symptoms similar to those of a panic or anxiety attack, including faintness, weakness, sweating, shakiness, hunger, anxiety, and more rarely, irritability and heart palpitations. Other symptoms may develop because the nervous system is being deprived of an essential energy source. These include headache, confusion, personality changes, muscle weakness, fatigue, and lack of coordination. Vision may become dim, blurry, or double, and in more severe reactions, seizures or unconsciousness may result" (Hypoglycemia, 2004, para. 5-6). Though this reaction is short-term and can be reversed, we want to ensure we prevent Hypoglycemia from happening.

Hyperglycemia is a beast. According to Alic, "Hyperglycemia is an abnormally high level of glucose (sugar) in the blood, which occurs when the body has too little insulin or cannot utilize insulin properly. Hyperglycemia is usually associated with diabetes mellitus, but transient Hyperglycemia can be caused by pregnancy, illness, injury, or other stresses. Prolonged Hyperglycemia can damage multiple organ systems. Hyperglycemia is also known as high blood sugar or high blood glucose" Alic 2017, para. 1). All in all, too much sugar can wreak havoc within the body, but the good news is we can control it with RX drugs, diet, and exercise. According to Alic, "The excess glucose overwhelms the kidneys, causing increased urination (osmotic diuresis), excess sugar in the urine (glycosuria), thirst, and dehydration. Because the body cannot utilize glucose, fats and proteins are broken down for energy, producing ketones as waste products that are excreted in the urine. In the absence of insulin, ketone build-up in the blood leads to diabetic ketoacidosis (DKA) and potentially to a life-threatening diabetic coma" (Alic 2017, para. 5). In the end, if we don't take control of Diabetes, the disorder will take control of us—and could even cause us to lose extremities, cause kidney failure, or even loss of eyesight.

According to Healthy Eating for T2D, "If Diabetes goes untreated or poorly treated, it can cause serious complications, such as vision loss, kidney damage, nerve damage, narrowing of blood vessels leading to amputations, etc. Nearly all complications develop from having high blood glucose levels over many years, with other factors such as high blood pressure contributing. Overall, the risk for death among people with diabetes is about twice that of people without Diabetes of a similar age" (Healthy Eating, para. 11, see Figure 2). You have the power to fight back and beat Diabetes; it starts with taking control of your diagnosis, it begins with understanding the disease. Like my neighbor Mike, once he knew better and grasped a better understanding of his diagnosis, he started eating, feeling, and living better. Awareness is the key!

Remember, pattern and habit rewire the brain. Neuroplasticity takes time but is inevitable once the body starts a new technique. The brain and the body will constantly adapt to change as long as the process isn't interrupted. We must do our part by watering and nourishing the seed—only then will you benefit from the results. Remember, nothing worth having ever came easy. "The seed you plant today is not the day you will eat the fruit" (Fabienne Fredrickson). So, stay true to your health and wellness routine and know that the results *will* follow. All in all, once we start eating healthier, increase activity levels, eliminate stressors, reduce or eliminate alcohol and cigarettes from our lives, and create a healthy environment to live and work—we will see and feel a positive transformation within ourselves. Trust the process; healing is on the other side of fear.

Impending Publication:

- The Placebo & Neuroplasticity: Beating Multiple Sclerosis (MS) with your Mind

References

Afaya, R. A., Bam, V., Azongo, T. B., & Afaya, A. (2020). Knowledge of chronic complications of Diabetes among persons living with type 2 diabetes mellitus in northern Ghana. *PloS One, 15*(10), e0241424. https://doi.org/10.1371/journal.pone.0241424 Retrieved from https://eds.a.ebscohost.com/eds/pdfviewer/pdfviewer?vid=29&sid=2da42c7 3-b198-4980-a4fa-3ab1a35bf1d4%40sdc-v-sessmgr02

Alic, M., & Mertz, L. (2017). Hyperglycemia. Gale (Ed.), *Gale virtual reference library: The Gale encyclopedia of nutrition and food labels*. Gale. Credo Reference: https://neumann.idm.oclc.org/login?url=https://search.credoreference.com/c ontent/entry/galegnafl/hyperglycemia/0?institutionId=6812

American Diabetes Association, (2021). *American diabetes association*, Retrieved from https://www.diabetes.org/resources/statistics/statistics-about-diabetes

Antioxidants (2019). In *The Gale Encyclopedia*. Retrieved from https://search-credoreference-com.neumann.idm.oclc.org/content/entry/galediets/antioxidants/0

Bernstein, H., & Bernstein, L. L. (2019). Type 2 diabetes in children: A growing problem. In Harvard Health Publications (Ed.), *Harvard Medical School commentaries on health*. Harvard Health Publications. Credo Reference: https://neumann.idm.oclc.org/login?url=https://search.credoreference.com/c ontent/entry/hhphoh/type_2_diabetes_in_children_a_growing_problem/0?in stitutionId=6812

Castorani, V., Polidori, N., Giannini, C., Blasetti, A., & Chiarelli, F. (2020).

Insulin resistance and type 2 diabetes in children. *Annals of Pediatric

Endocrinology & Metabolism, 25*(4), 217–226.

https://doi.org/10.6065/apem.2040090.045 Retrieved from

https://eds.a.ebscohost.com/eds/pdfviewer/pdfviewer?vid=12&sid=b4061fe5

-d136-4d02-9b36-82ea86976da5%40sdc-v-sessmgr03

CDC (2018). All About your A1C. *Center for Disease Control.* Retrieved from

https://www.cdc.gov/diabetes/managing/managing-blood-

sugar/a1c.html#:~:text=A%20normal%20A1C%20level%20is,for%20devel

oping%20type%202%20diabetes.

CDC & Prevention, (2021). About Chronic Diseases. *Center for Disease Control

and Prevention.* Retrieved from

https://www.cdc.gov/chronicdisease/about/index.htm

Healthy Eating for Type 2 Diabetes. (2019). In Harvard Medical School

(Ed.), *Harvard Medical School special health reports.* Harvard Health

Publications. Credo Reference:

https://neumann.idm.oclc.org/login?url=https://search.credoreference.com/c

ontent/entry/hhpharvard/healthy_eating_for_type_2_diabetes/0?institutionId

=6812

Health Line (2021). Diabetes Home Test Explained. *Health Line.* Retrieved from

https://www.healthline.com/health/diabetes/home-tests

Hypoglycemia. (2004). In K. J. Carlson, S. A. Eisenstat, & T. D. Ziporyn, *New

Harvard guide to women's health, the.* Harvard University Press. Credo

Reference:

https://neumann.idm.oclc.org/login?url=https://search.credoreference.com/c

ontent/entry/hupwh/hypoglycemia/0?institutionId=6812

Khan, G. I. (2008). Diabetes. In C. N. Svendsen, & A. D. Ebert, *Encyclopedia of stem cell research*. Sage Publications. Credo Reference: https://neumann.idm.oclc.org/login?url=https://search.credoreference.com/content/entry/sagestemcell/diabetes/0?institutionId=6812

Medical News Today, (2021). How can Antioxidants Benefit our Health? Retrieved from https://www.medicalnewstoday.com/articles/is-watermelon-keto#watermelon-nutrient-profile

Ratnesh, Shivaprasad, K. S., Kannan, S., Khadilkar, K. S., Sravani, G. V., & Raju, R. (2020). Identifying the Burden and Predictors of Diabetes Distress among Adult Type 2 Diabetes Mellitus Patients. *Indian Journal of Community Medicine*, *45*(4), 497–500. https://doi.org/10.4103/ijcm.IJCM_533_19 Retrieved from https://eds.a.ebscohost.com/eds/detail/detail?vid=21&sid=2da42c73-b198-4980-a4fa-3ab1a35bf1d4%40sdc-v-sessmgr02&bdata=JkF1dGhUeXBlPXNzbyZzaXRlPWVkcy1saXZlJnNjb3BlPXNpdGU%3d#AN=146717423&db=ccm

What Causes Diabetes? Find out and take control (2021). *American Diabetes Association*. Retrieved from https://www.diabetes.org/diabetes-risk

Yi-Jen Fang, Tien-Yuan Wu, Jung-Nien Lai, Cheng-Li Lin, Ni Tien, & Yun-Ping Lim (2021). Association between Depression, Antidepression Medications, and the Risk of Developing Type 2 Diabetes Mellitus: A Nationwide Population-Based Retrospective Cohort Study in Taiwan. *BioMed Research International*, *2021*, 1–10. https://doi.org/10.1155/2021/8857230 Retrieved from https://eds.a.ebscohost.com/eds/detail/detail?vid=13&sid=2da42c73-b198-4980-a4fa-3ab1a35bf1d4%40sdc-v-

Dear Reader,

My name is Vanessa B. Jackson, AKA Sister Moon. I would like to thank you for reading my brief book regarding Type 2 diabetes. I hope you found the information useful and insightful. For all things Sister Moon, please search my website SisterMoonYoga.Net for the latest health & wellness information, yoga and mindfulness classes, and so much more.

Note to self:
Use the following sections to write personal notes

Note to Self:

Healthy Eating Tips:

What Makes me Feel Good: Do more of that!

Who is Supportive: Spend more time with them!

Goals & Visions:

Situations that no longer serve me: What did I outgrow:

What can I do to boost my happiness:

When I was younger, I always wanted to:

Note to self: Everything and everyone doesn't deserve a response: Why is this so?

What situations and circumstances aren't ideal for my future:

Self-affirmation: "I will not entertain anyone or anything that doesn't benefit my future self."

The ability to change comes from within—as does sincere happiness. We hold the power to create a new life for ourselves. If we want different results—and if we're going to attract positive outcomes—we must first feel, be, and think differently.

Remember, we must "be the energy we want to attract" (Gandhi).

"Be the change" (Mahatma Gandhi)

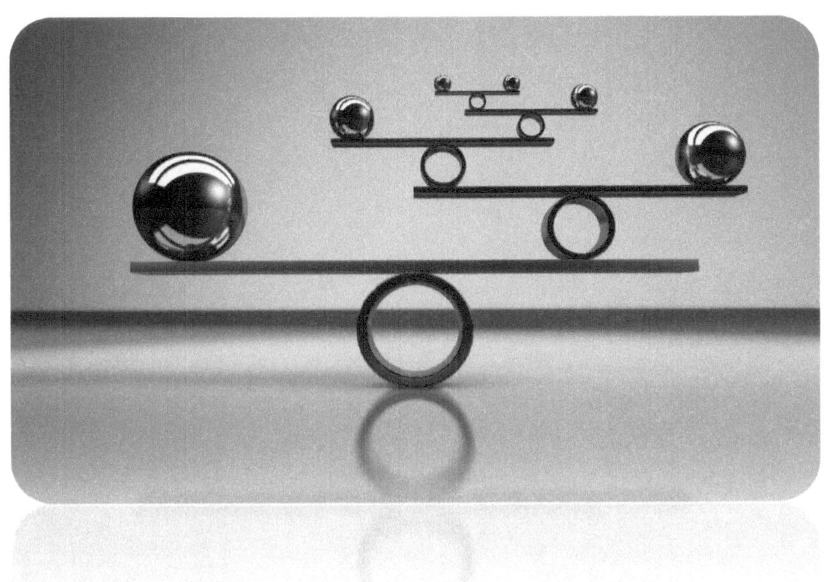